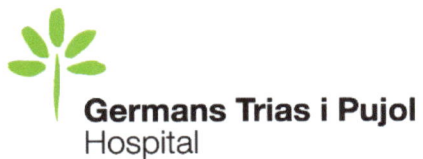
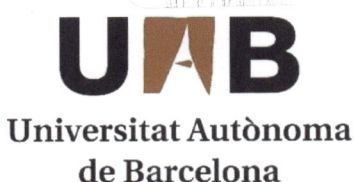

ANATOMY FOR TRANSORAL APPROACHES IN OROPHARYNGEAL SURGERY

Authors:

David Virós Porcuna. MD. Phd.
ENT- Head & Neck Surgeon. Hospital Universitari Germans Trias i Pujol. Badalona. Barcelona.

Rosa M. Mirapeix Lucas. MD. Phd.
Professor of Human Anatomy Department.
Universidad Autónoma de Barcelona.

Constanza Viña Soria. MD.
ENT- Head & Neck Surgeon. Hospital Universitari Germans Trias i Pujol. Badalona. Barcelona.

Carlos Pollán Guisasola. MD.
ENT- Head & Neck Surgeon.
Head of Department. Hospital Universitari Germans Trias i Pujol. Badalona. Barcelona.

Mar Palau Viarnès. MD.
ENT- Head & Neck Surgeon. Hospital Universitari Germans Trias i Pujol. Badalona. Barcelona.

Laura Pardo Muñoz. MD.
ENT- Head & Neck Surgeon. Hospital Universitari Germans Trias i Pujol. Badalona. Barcelona.

Abbreviations

SCm	Superior Constrictor muscle
MCm	Middle Constrictor muscle
SPm	Stylopharyngeus muscle
SGm	Styloglossus muscle
SHm	Stylohyoid muscle
GPm	Glossopharyngeus muscle
HGm	Hyoglossus muscle
PGm	Palatoglossus muscle
PPm	Palatopharyngeus muscle
pbDGm	Posterior belly of the digastric muscle.

Index

Introduction	9
Chapter 1- Oropharyngeal Lateral Wall Dissection	**13**
First layer	13
Second layer	18
Third layer	22
Chapter 2- Base of the Tongue Dissection	**25**
Chapter 3- Oropharyngeal Lateral Wall Endoscopic Dissection	**29**
First layer	29
Second layer	33
Third layer	38
Chapter 4- Base of the Tongue Endoscopic Dissection	**43**

INTRODUCTION

Over the last decades, oropharyngeal cancer treatment has changed due to the introduction of new surgical techniques such as transoral approaches. These new techniques provide oncological results that are comparable to previous treatment but with shorter hospital stays and the preservation of functions.

This surgery makes necessary to understand the anatomy of the upper aerodigestive pathway from the inside-out, as opposed to the inverse, which is the way head and neck surgeons have classically understood it. Although descriptions of the anatomy from medial to lateral have been published, a clear anatomic stratification of this area should help in the planning and execution of this surgery.

This book is the basic guide for an anatomical course with the purpose to identify anatomic landmarks in the oropharynx and base of the tongue. This can help surgeons identify neurovascular elements of the surgical field during transoral robotic surgery quickly and accurately.

The Hands-on Course TransOral Approaches in Oropharyngeal Surgery is a practical course, where the trainee will dissect the lateral wall of the oropharynx and the base of the tongue in an formalin-fixed head and a fresh cadaveric head.

The dissection in the formalin-fixed cadaver will be performed, in a sagittal sectioned head, with the help of optical magnification either by means of magnifying glasses or a surgical microscope.

In the fresh cadaveric head, two trainees will perform an endoscopic dissection, using three and four-hand techniques. A 10 mm straight endoscope and dissection material will be used. Furthermore, dissection work will also be done through a Da Vinci Xi type robotic surgery platform by all the trainees over two fresh heads.

The cadaveric head will be located in a surgical position. Davis-Boyle and Feith-Kastelbauer mouth gag modified by Weinstein and O'Malley will be used.

The objective of this course is the anatomical description of the structures located in the lateral wall of the oropharynx and base of the tongue in the direction from the inside to the outside and in layers that can help the planning of transoral surgery. It is important to remember that this is not a course of surgery but of surgical anatomy. It will be the anatomical dissection that sets the work guidelines and not the surgical technique strictly.

The lateral oropharyngeal wall is divided into 3 layers from medial to lateral, based in the styloid muscle diaphragm. The first layer, medial to constrictor muscles. The second layer, medial to styloid muscles. The third layer, lateral to styloid diaphragm.

This clasification is considered to help the planning of surgical resection as well as to plan the need for an associated reconstructive procedure.

For the dissection of the lateral wall of the oropharynx, the following limits have been considered: anterior limit, retromolar trigone and anterior tonsillar pillar; posterior boundary, the pharynx; upper limit, the styloid process; lower limit, the major horn of the hyoid bone and as a lateral limit, the medial pterygoid muscle.

For the base of tongue dissection, the lingual tonsil has been considered as the anterior limit; the epiglottis as a posterior limit; the glossosepiglottic ligament as a medial limit, and finally the medial pterygoid muscle as a lateral limit.

OROPHARYNGEAL LATERAL WALL DISSECTION

FIRST LAYER.

The first layer extends from the mucosa of the oropharynx to the constrictor muscles. Before starting the dissection, we will identify the following anatomical structures from anterior to posterior: the anterior tonsillar pillar, the palatine tonsil, the posterior tonsillar pillar and the pharyngoepiglottic fold. We will proceed to the extraction of the mucosa taking into account that the mucosa is very attached to the deeper plane. We will perform a tonsillectomy and identify the fascial layer that protects the constrictor muscles (Fig. 1).

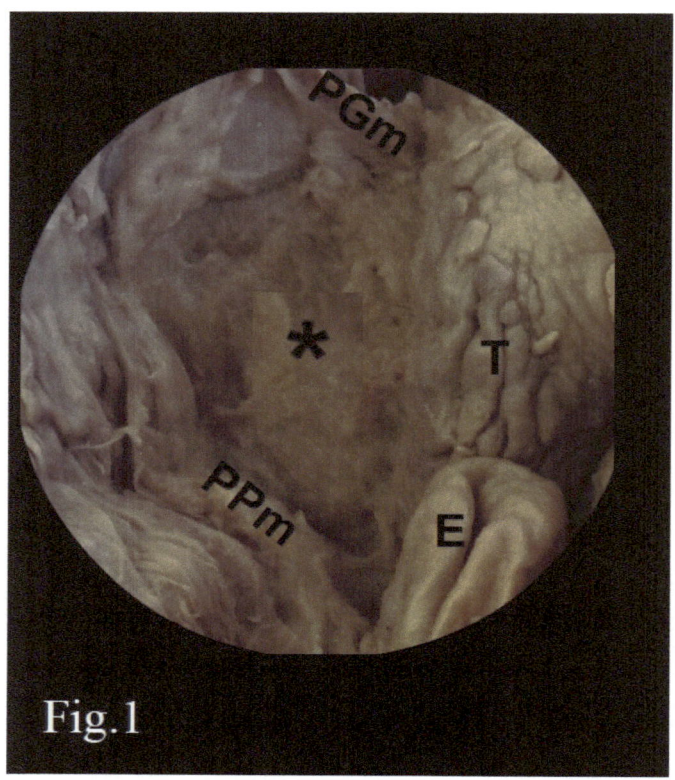

Fig 1: Lateral wall of the oropharynx, left side. We can see the fascia (*) over the constrictor muscles . E, Epiglotis; T, Tongue; PPm, Palatopharyngeus muscle; PGm, Palatoglossus muscle

We will clean the area in order to identify the following muscle elements: the palatoglossus muscle (PGm), the superior constrictor muscle (SCm), the middle constrictor muscle (MCm) and the palatopharyngeus muscle (PPm). Sometimes it is difficult to differentiate one constrictor muscle from another due to the presence of multiple muscle bands between them. For this reason, we will look at the fibers orientation. The SCm has horizontal fibers and overlaps the MCm which has a post-superior direction. While mCS is related to PGm, MCm is related to PPm, often lacing its fibers.

In this layer we will observe the tonsillar vascular network. The upper branches come from the descending palatine artery (maxillary artery branch), the ascending palatine artery (facial artery branch) and the ascending pharyngeal artery (external carotid artery branch). The middle branches proceed from the facial artery and the lower part of the tonsillar fossa is irrigated by branches of the lingual artery. In general, the lingual branches are larger than the facial branches and enter the tonsillar bed through the glossosepiglottic space (Fig. 2). Constantly, there is a slightly vascularized area located at the level of the lingual insertion of the PGm.

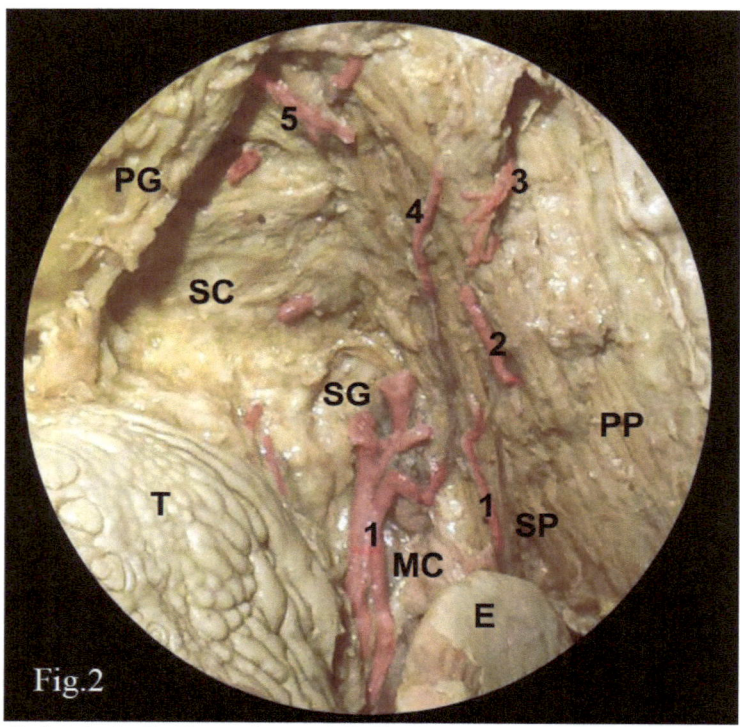

Fig 2: Lateral wall of the oropharynx, right side. We can see the the arteries of the tonsilar fossa coming from the descending palatine artery (1), ascending palatine (2), and ascending pharyngeal (3), facial (4) and lingual (5). E, Epiglotis; T, Tongue; SCm, Superior Constrictor muscle;MCm, Middle Constrictor muscle ;SGm, Styloglossus muscle; PPm, Palatopharyngeus muscle; PGm, Palatoglossus muscle.

At the junction of the SCm and the MCm, a space between 1 and 3 cm appears where the lingual branch of the glossopharyngeal nerve emerges. If this space is wide, the styloglossus muscle (SGm) can be distinguished at the bottom of it (Fig. 3).

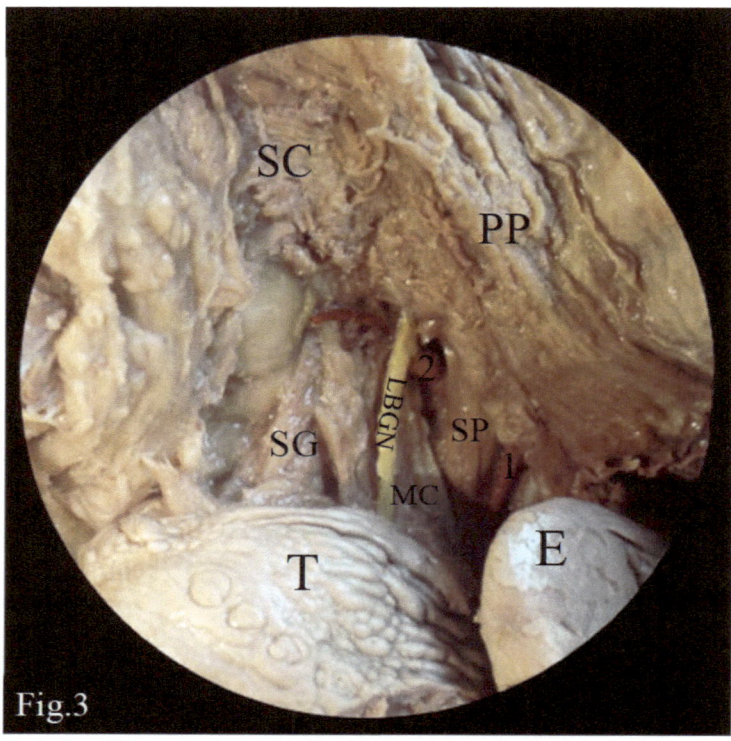

Fig 3: Constrictors muscles, right side of the oropharynx. E, Epiglotis; T, Tongue; SCm, Superior Constrictor muscle; MCm, Middle Constrictor muscle ;SGm, Styloglossus muscle; PPm, Palatopharyngeus muscle; PGm, Palatoglossus muscle; LBIX, lingual branch of the glossopharyngeal nerve.

SECOND LAYER.

In order to reach the second layer, the SCm and the MCm must be sectioned, then oropharyngeal fascia appears. When this fascia is removed, we can identify the muscular and neurovascular structures located in the parapharyngeal space surrounded and protected by fat. We will first identify the SGm and proceed to dissect it upwards until it reaches the styloid process. We will observe the full extent of SGm from its styloid origin to its lingual insertion.

The SGm is the most anterior (ventral) muscle and the shortest of the three styloid muscles. At this level, we will locate the stylopharyngeus muscle (SPm) intersecting with SGm fibers. As they move towards their lower insertion points, both muscles separate from each other. The SPm is the most medial and posterior of all styloid muscles. It descends first covered by the SCm (lateral to it) and then in its lower third it is located between the SCm and the MCm, going parallel to the anterior border of the PPm for lower insertion.

Parallel to the SPm runs the stylohyoid ligament, a fibrous cord that descends from the tip of the styloid process to the hyoid bone. Lateral and parallel to the stylohyoid ligament, the stylohyoid muscle (SHm) and the posterior belly of the digastric muscle (pbDGm) can be identified (Fig. 4).

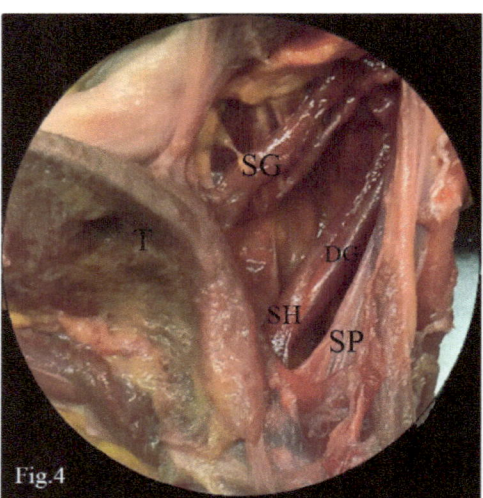 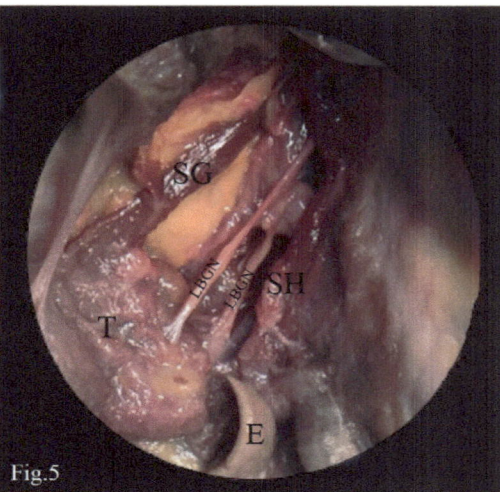

Fig 4: View of the right side of the oropharynx after section of constrictor muscles. T, Tongue; SGm, Styloglossus muscle; SPm, Stylopharyngeus muscle; SHm, Stylohyoid muscle; pbDGm, posterior belly of Digastric muscle.

Fig 5: View of the right side of the oropharynx after section of constrictor muscles. We can see the glossopharyngeal nerve (IXn) and his lingual branches. T, Tongue; E, Epiglotis; SGm, Styloglossus muscle; SHm, Stylohyoid muscle.

In the first layer we identified the lingual branches of the glossopharyngeal nerve. Once we have sectioned the SCm and the MCm, we can see these branches standing between SGm and SHm (Fig. 5).

If we continue the dissection upwards we will find the glossopharyngeal nerve trunk, medial to the styloid process. From here, the glossopharyngeal nerve descends on the lateral surface of the SPm in its upper third, more distally medializes and gives its muscular branches. It is then placed between the SHm and the SGm (Fig. 5). At this level it gives its lingual branches that reach the tongue medially to the

MCm (Fig. 3). The glossopharyngeal nerve is in the same layer as the styloid musculature (SGm, SPm and SHm).

In this layer we can identify the arteries that will arise the tonsillar vascularization. Thus, in the upper half we will identify the ascending and descending palatine arteries and the ascending pharyngeal artery. Medial to SHm we can observe the facial artery giving the middle tonsil branches (Fig. 6). In the lower part we will find the lingual artery. Sometimes it is necessary to cut the stylohyoid ligament to observe the artery. At this point we can observe how the pbDGm crosses the lingual artery from lateral to medial.

THIRD LAYER

Lateral to the styloid muscles, the parapharyngeal space muscles appears. This space is in continuity with the submandibular space through a communication, limited laterally by the medial pterygoid muscle and medially by the SGm and SCm. The lateral wall of the parapharyngeal space is made up of the medial pterygoid muscle with its fascia, the ascending branch of the jaw and the submandibular gland (inferolateral to SGm and inferoposterior to SHm and pbDGm).

The SGm is an important anatomical landmark for the location of parapharyngeal space's neurovascular structures. Lateral to the SGm we can identify the external carotid artery that will raise the lingual and facial branches at this level, as well as the internal carotid artery (Fig. 6). The facial and lingual veins will follow the arteries path, placing themselves in a more lateral plane, to drain into the internal jugular vein.

Anterior to the joint between the pharyngoepiglottic fold and the epiglottis, the upper branch of the superior laryngeal artery appears along with the internal branch of the superior laryngeal nerve.

In this layer we can see the whole extension of glossopharyngeal nerve. Posterior to it we can identify the superior laryngeal nerve. The pharyngeal branch of the vagus nerve crosses the glossopharyngeal nerve or, less frequently, runs parallel to innervate the pharyngeal wall (Fig. 6).

Expanding the dissection inferior and anterior to SGm, the lingual nerve can be distinguished between the lingual surface of the jaw and the lateral surface of the medial pterygoid muscle.

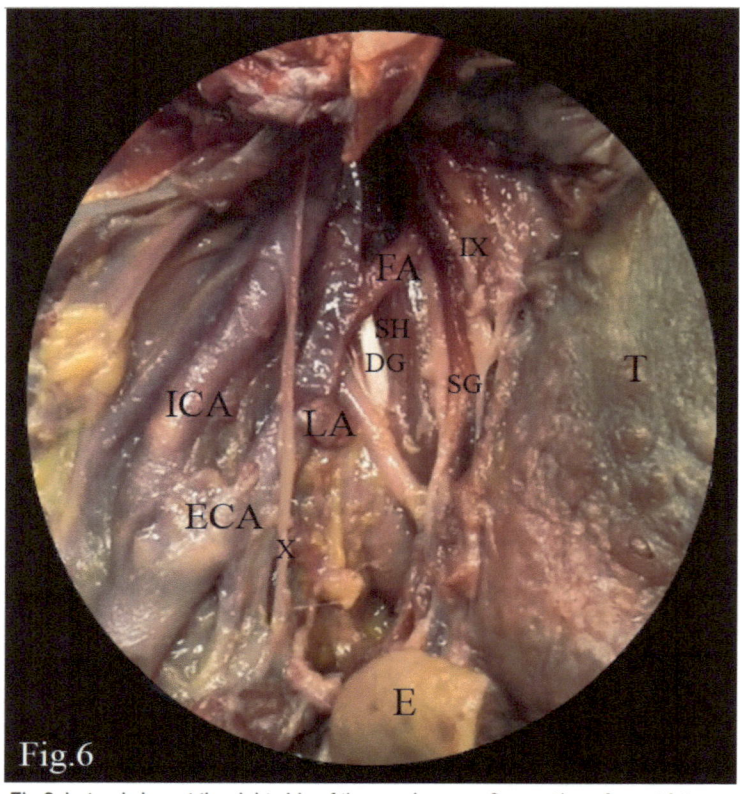

Fig 6: Lateral view ot the right side of the oropharynx after section of constrictor and styloid muscles. ICa, internal carotid artery; Fa, Facial artery; La, Lingual artery; E, Epiglotis; T, Tongue; Lv, lingual vein; IJv, Internal Jugular vein; IXn, Glossopharyngeal nerve; Xn, Vagus nerve.

BASE OF TONGUE DISSECTION

We will first identify the superficial landmarks: the lateral and medial glossoepiglottic folds, the pharyngoepiglottic fold and the lingual "V".

Approximately in the middle of pharyngoepiglottic fold in depth, the greater horn of the hyoid bone will be located. We will observe how the midpoint of this fold corresponds to the upper part of the epiglottis. Then we can start with the mucosa excision. First, we will find the MCm, lateral to this muscle and medial to the hyoglossus muscle (HGm) we can locate the lingual artery. After its origin, the artery describes an upper turn and it is directed towards the tongue parallel to the greater horn of the hyoid bone. At this level it is related to the pbDGm (Fig 7.8).

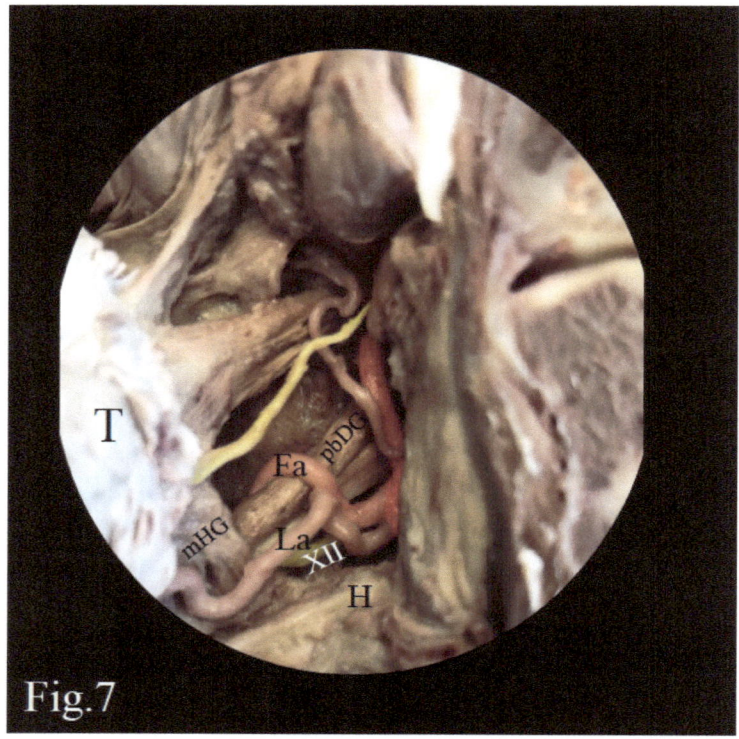

Fig 7: Far lateral view ot the right side of the oropharynx after section of constrictor. La, Lingual artery; Fa, Facial Artery; H, Hyoid bone; T, Tongue; HGm, Hyoglossus muscle; pbDG, posterior belly of the Digastric muscle; XII, hypoglossal nerve.

The lingual artery on its way to the tongue is located inferior to the SGm, before dividing into its terminal branches: the deep lingual artery and the sublingual. This artery can be followed at its entrance to the tongue until its division into the lingual dorsal branch.

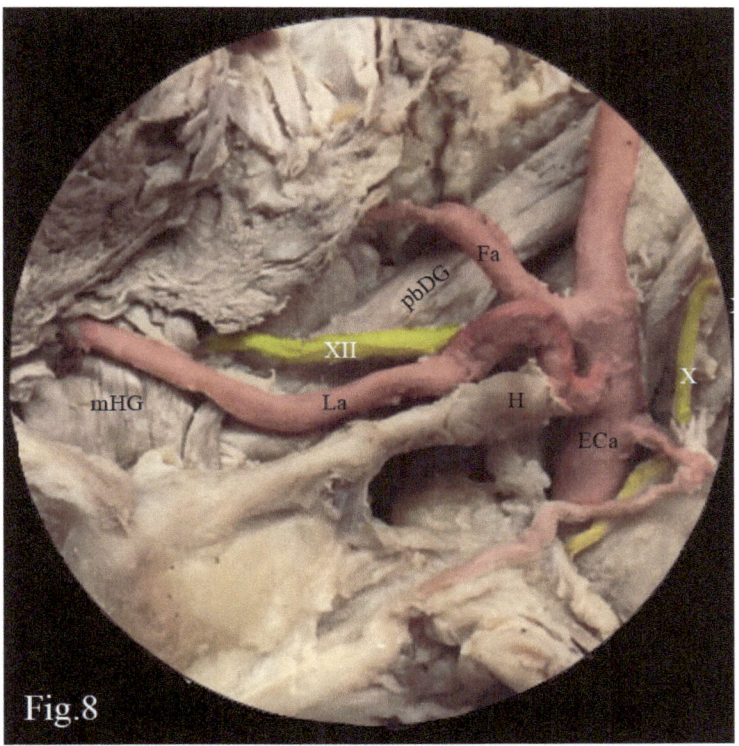

Fig 8: Right base of tongue. ECa, external carotid artery; Fa, Facial artery; La, Lingual artery; H, Hyoid bone; HGm, Hyoglossus muscle; X, Vagus nerve; XII, Hypoglossal nerve; pbDG, posterior belly of the Digastric muscle.

The mHG separates the lingual artery from the hypoglossal nerve, being the artery medial and the nerve lateral (Fig. 8). At this level the hypoglossal nerve is accompanied by the lingual veins (Fig. 8).

Lower and posterior to the greater hyoid horn we will identify the superior laryngeal nerve and artery.

OROPHARYNGEAL LATERAL WALL ENDOSCOPIC DISSECTION

FIRST LAYER.

The first step is to identify the following structures of the oropharynx: anterior and posterior pillars, tonsillar fossa, soft palate and posterior pharyngeal wall (Fig. 9).

We will also locate the pharyngoepiglottic folds, the glossoepiglottic medial and lateral folds.

We then proceed to the excision of the mucosa of the soft palate, anterior pillar and retromolar trigone. A tonsillectomy will be performed.

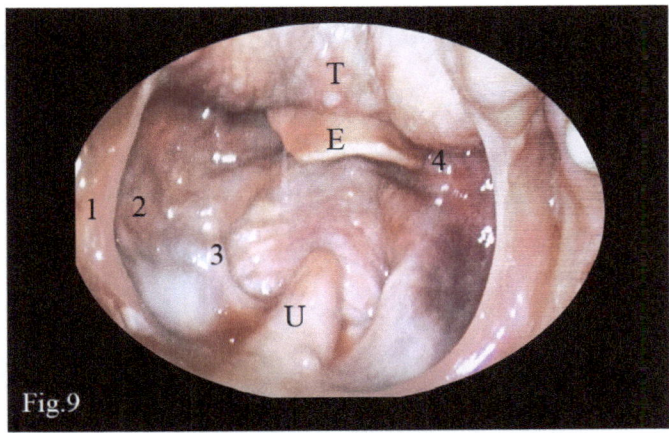

Fig 9: Endoscopic view of the oropharynx. E, Epiglotis; T, Base of Tongue; U, Uvula; 1, Anterior Tonsillar Pillar; 2, Tonsillar Fossa; 3, Posterior Tonsillar Pillar; 4, Pharyngoepiglotic fold.

The arteries that supply the tonsillar fossa accompanied by concomitant veins will be identified. These arteries will reach the tonsil after perforating the constrictor muscles.

The superior arteries, accompanied by their concomitant veins, reach the tonsillar bed after perforating the SCm. The inferior tonsil arteries come from the facial and lingual arteries and reach the tonsillar bed after perforating the MCm (Fig 10).

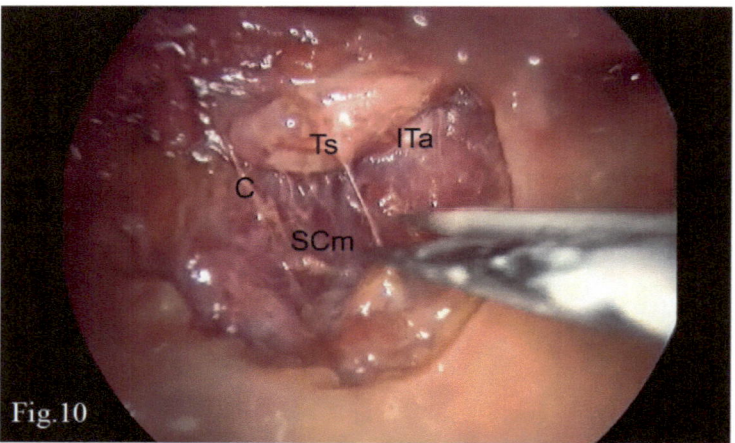

Fig 10: Lateral wall, right oropharynx. Ts, tonsil; C, Tonsillar capsula; SCm, Superior Constrictor muscle; ITa, Inferior Tonsillar artery.

Exposure of the upper and middle constrictor muscles is performed. The fibers of the SCm are placed horizontally, while those of the MCm have a postero-superior direction. Its palatine origin frequently appears mixed with the PPm without a clear dissection plane between them.

At this point the lingual branch of the glossopharyngeal nerve can be located between the SCm and the MCm, which corresponds roughly to the midpoint between the PGm and the PPm (Fig 11).

Here there is a variable size space where we can identify the SGm at the bottom of it. The lingual branch of the glossopharyngeal nerve is posteroinferior to the SGm.

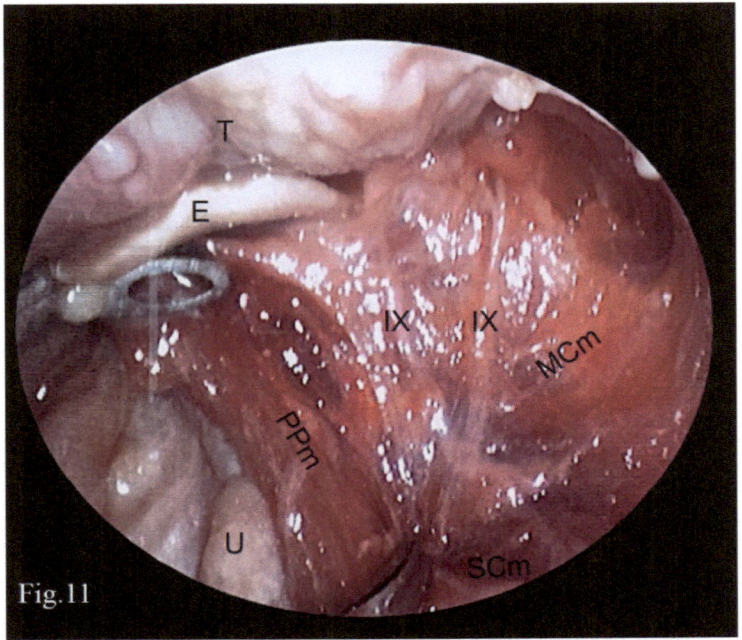

Fig 11: Lateral wall, right oropharynx. U, Uvula; E, Epiglotis; T, Base of Tongue; T, tonsil; SCm, Superior Constrictor muscle; MCm, Middle Constrictor muscle; IX, lingual branches of Glossopharyngeal nerve; PPm, Palatopharyngeus muscle.

SECOND LAYER.

The next step is to remove the constrictor muscles. Here it is recommended to follow the PPm medially until identify the prevertebral fascia. Here we can find the fat from the parapharyngeal space and the pharyngeal vascular plexus (Fig 12).

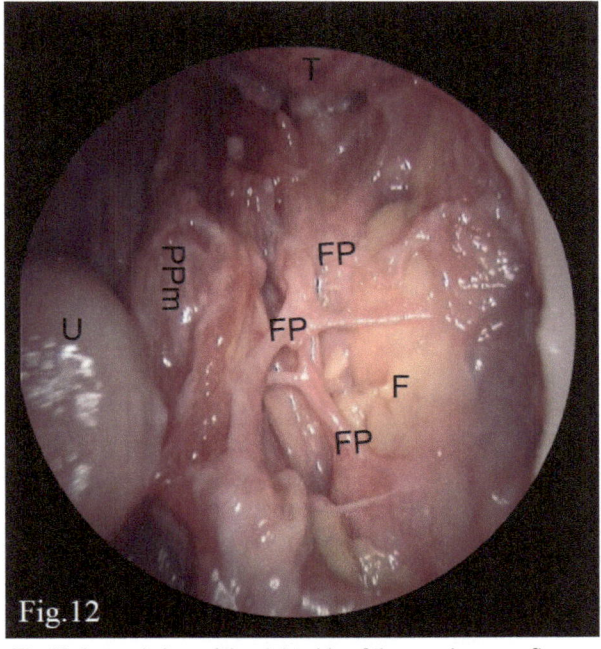

Fig 12: Lateral view of the right side of the oropharynx after section of constrictor muscles. PPm, Palatopharyngeus muscle; U, Uvula; T, Tongue; FP, Pharyngeal vascular Plexus; F, Fat from the parapharyngeal space.

If this dissection is initiated between the SCm and MCm, the SGm is easily identified and can be dissected in the superior direction to the styloid process.

Fat is removed from the parapharyngeal space to expose the styloid diaphragm. We will observe how SGm and SPm overlap at the level of the styloid process and separate as they descend.

The SPm is the most medial muscle of this diaphragm. Its upper part is located lateral to the SCm and once it reaches the lower edge of this muscle is placed parallel to the lower edge of the PPm (Fig 13).

We proceed to follow in cranial direction the lingual branch of the glossopharyngeal nerve, from the initial identification point (in the first layer) to the styloid process. The glossopharyngeal nerve will be located medial to SHm and lateral to SGm (Fig 13).

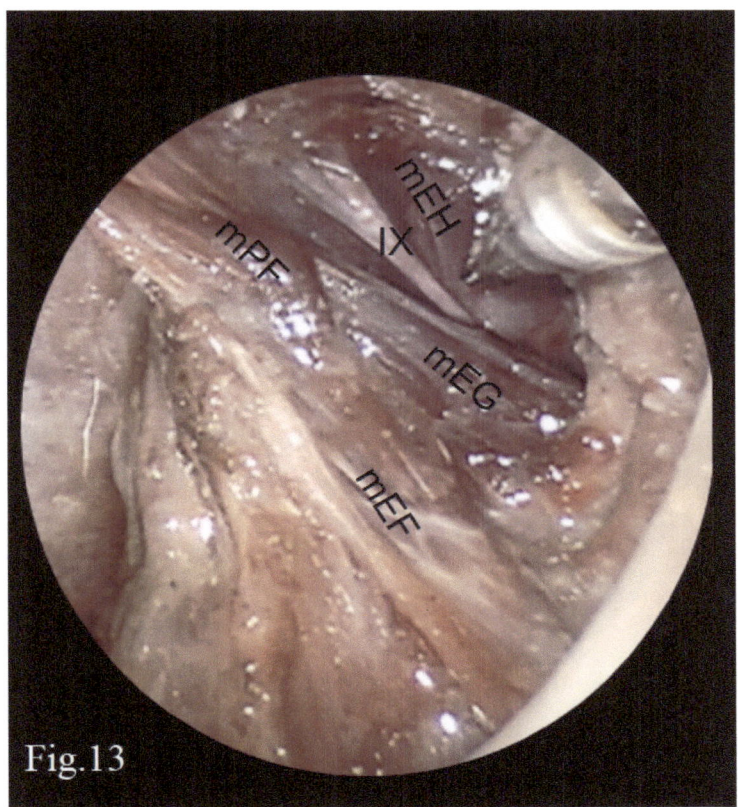

Fig 13: Lateral view of the right side of the oropharynx after section of constrictor muscles. SCm, Superior Constrictor muscle; SGm, Styloglossus muscle; IXn, glossopharyngeal nerve; SPm, Stylopharyngeus muscle; PPm, Palatopharyngeus muscle (partially resected).

At this point, the glossopharyngeal nerve turns posterior to the SPm, standing lateral to this muscle. Here the nerve gives branches for this muscle, the posterior pharyngeal wall and the carotid branches.

Parallel and lateral to the SPm runs the stylohyoid ligament, a fibrous cord that descends from the tip of the styloid process to the hyoid bone. Lateral and parallel to the stylohyoid ligament, SHm can be identified with pbDGm. The pbDGm is located lateral to the external carotid artery. This artery is identified when dissection is performed between SPm and SGm (Fig 14).

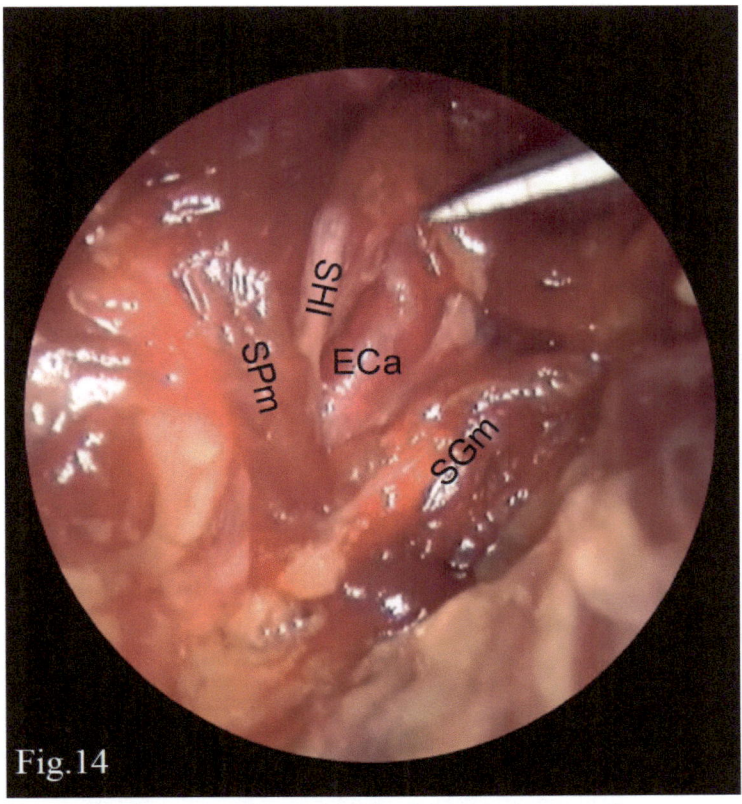

Fig 14: Caudal area of the right side of the oropharynx after dissection between Stylopharyngeus and Styloglossus muscles. SPm, Stylopharyngeus muscle; SGm, Styloglossus muscle; SHl, Stylohyoid ligament; ECa, External Carotid artery.

In this second layer, muscle structures will keep in situ.

The lingual artery is located laterally to the lower third of the mEG. We can find here its third portion before entering the base of the tongue and giving its dorsal branches. If the most lateral portion of the stylohyoid ligament is cut, the second portion of the lingual artery can be exposed, when it is located superiorly to the greater hyoid horn.

Above the upper half of the mEH, the facial artery is identified medially crossing it.

THIRD LAYER.

This layer is located lateral to the styloid diaphragm. The SGm continues to be an important landmark in this layer, especially for vascular structures.

Lateral to styloid muscles, in the lateral wall of the parapharyngeal space, the medial pterygoid muscle with its fascia and the mandibular ramus are identified (Fig 15).

Lateral to the SGm we can identify the external carotid artery that will give the lingual and facial branches at this level (Fig 16).

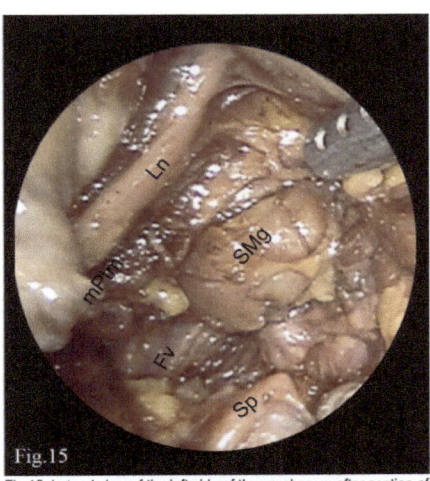

Fig 15: Lateral view of the left side of the oropharynx after section of styloid muscles. Ln, Lingual nerve; mPtm, medial Pterygoid muscle; SMg, submaxilar gland; Fv, Facial vein; Sp, Styloid process.

The parapharyngeal space is in continuity with the submandibular space by a communication, limited laterally by the pterygoid medially and medially by the SGm and the SCm

39

The submandibular gland is located inferolateral to SGm and inferoposterior to SHm and pbDGm.

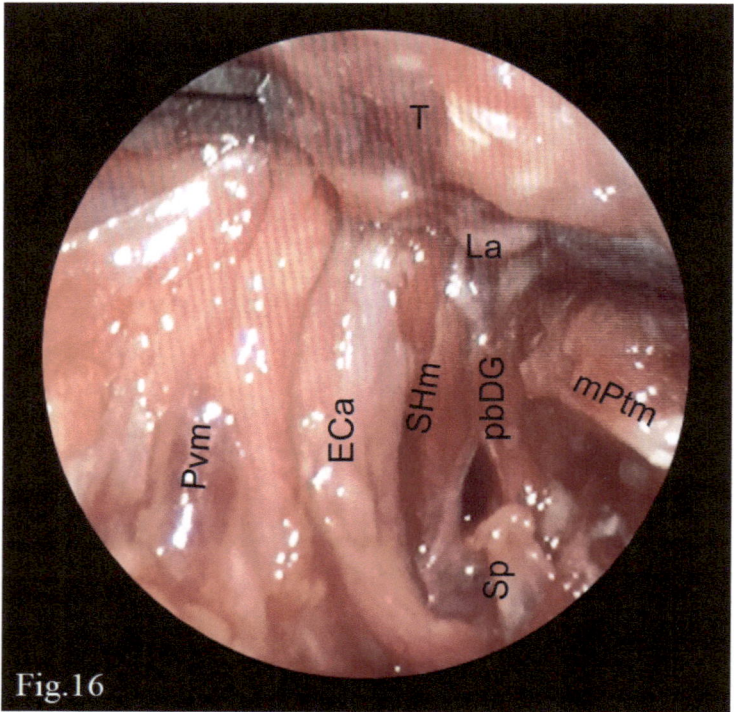

Fig.16

Fig 16: Right side of the oropharynx after ressection of Stylopharyngeus and Styloglossus muscles. Pvm, prevertebral muscles; S ECa, External Carotid artery; SGm, Styloglossus muscle; SHm, Stylohyoid muscle; Sp, Styloid process; pbDG, Posterior belly of digastric muscle; La, Lingual artery; T, base of Tongue; mPtm, medial Pterygoid muscle.

The lingual artery is located lateral and posterior to the SGm in its lower third, while in this same plane at the upper level is the facial artery crossing medial to the pbDGm and the SHm.

Next, the SPm and SGm will be removed (Fig 16).

The internal carotid artery is located posterolateral to the SGm, in a triangle formed by SGm, SPm and the stylohyoid ligament.

The pharyngeal branch of the vagus nerve crosses medially to the ICA and posterior to the hypoglossal nerve in this third plane (Fig 17).

Variations in the course and relation to the

oropharynx of the internal and external carotid arteries are not rare, 10% to 40% and up to 8%, respectively.

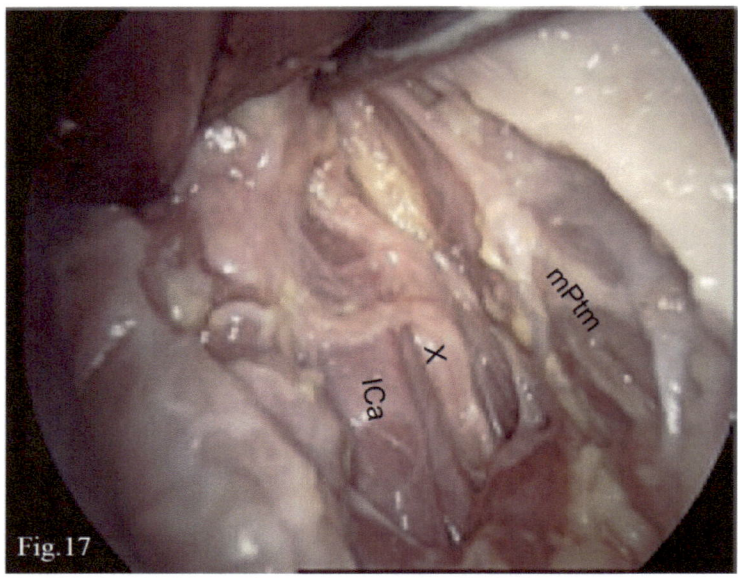

Fig 17: Right side of the oropharynx after ressection of Stylopharyngeus and Styloglossus muscles. mPtm, medial Pterygoid muscle; X, vagus nerve; ICa, Internal Carotid artery.

BASE OF TONGUE ENDOSCOPIC DISSECTION

The complete exposure of the tongue base, as well as the work on it, may be difficult because of the mouth gag used and cephalometric head characteristics. The main objective of this dissection will be the identification of the neurovascular structures of vital importance in this area.

The initial work will be on the lateral area for the identification of the entrance of the neurovascular pedicle. Initially, the superficial landmarks must be recognized in order to carry out dissection work in this area: medial and lateral glossoepiglottic folds, the pharyngoepiglottic fold and the lingual V.

The central base of tongue contains lymphoid tissue until it reaches the deep muscles (genioglossus and geniohyoid).

The tip of the greater horn of hyoid bone is located in the pharyngoepiglottic fold, lateral to the free edge of the epiglottis approximately at the midpoint of the fold. This is an important reference in tongue base surgery.

Inferior and posterior to it, the internal branch of the superior

laryngeal nerve, the superior thyroid artery, and the carotid bifurcation can be located (Fig. 18).

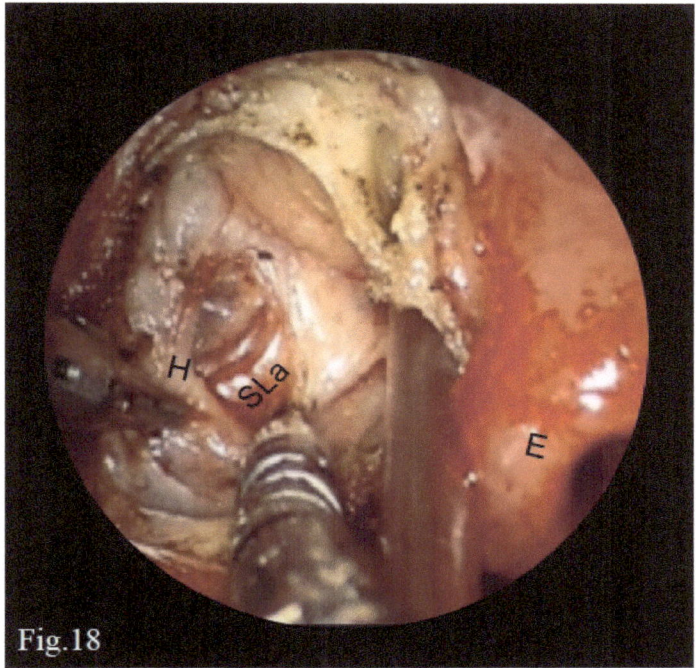

Fig 18: Caudal area, left side, 3rd plane. E, epiglotis; SLa, Superior Laryngeal artery; H, Hyoid bone.

Superior to the tip of the greater horn of the hyoid, the hypoglossal nerve and lingual artery can be identified, with lingual artery being the closest to the bone

Although significant variability in the origin of the lingual artery has been reported, its relation to the greater horn of the hyoid bone is relatively constant.

The lingual artery is located in the triangle formed by the HGm, the SGm and the greater hyoid horn (Fig. 19).

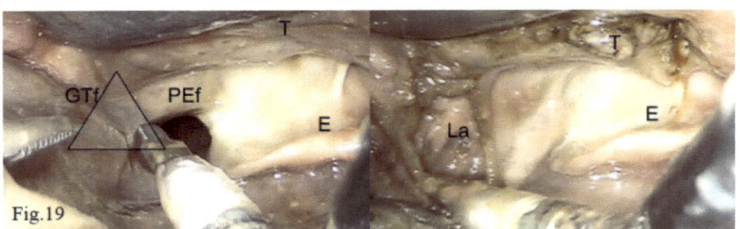

Fig 19: Base of tongue, left side. Identification of the lingual artery. E, epiglotis; T, base of Tongue; PEf, PharyngoEpiglotic fold; GTf, GlossoTonsillar fold.

To reach this artery we suggest to start the dissection at the junction between pharyngoepiglottic fold and glossotonsillar fold.

Once the mucosa and submucosa of the area are removed, the lower third of the SHm is found. Then the dissection proceeds mobilizating superomedially this muscle and the first segment of the lingual artery appears.

The HGm forms the lateral margin of the lingual artery. Once this muscle is medialized the hypoglossal nerve is identified(Fig 20).

The lingual artery can be followed at its entrance to the base of the tongue, between the genioglossus muscle and the tongue, until the division in the lingual dorsal branch. The dorsal branch is never found posterior to the line formed by the lingual V. This artery becomes superficial in the anterior area and lateral to the lingual V. No significant vascularization is found at the midline level of the tongue.

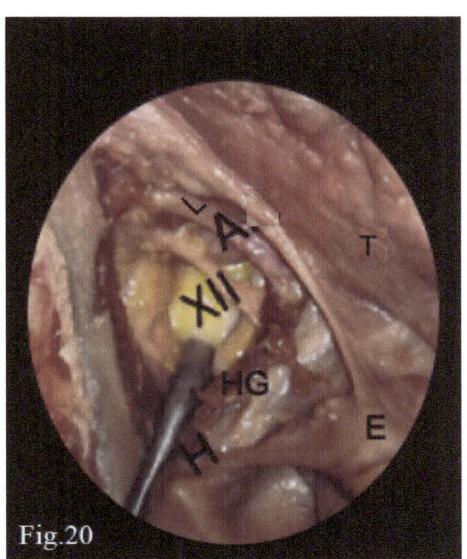

Fig 20: Base of tongue, left side, after ressection of hyoglossus muscle. T, base of Tongue; LA, Lingual artery; E, epiglotis; H, Hyod bone; HG, Hyoglossus muscle; XII, hypoglossal nerve.

Table: Anatomic Stratification of the Lateral Wall of the Oropharynx

Layer	Landmarks	Muscles	Vessels	Nerves	Other Structures
First	PGm	PGm	Tonsillar branches from	Lingual branch of the IX n	Tonsils
	PPm	PPm	Ascending palatine a		Tonsillar capsule
		SGm	Descending palatine a		Fascial layer
		SCm	Ascending pharyngeal a		
		MCm	Facial a		
			Lingual a		
			Tonsillar veins		
Second	Styloid muscles	SGm	Vessels that supply tonsils	Lingual branch of the IX n	Buccopharyngeal fascia
	SGm	SPm	Pharyngeal venous plexus		Stylohyoid ligament
	SPm	SHm	Lingual artery	IX n	
	SHm	pbDGm	Facial artery	XII n	
Third	SGm	Medial pterygoid	Internal carotid artery	Lingual n	Mandibular ramus
	SPm	SGm	External carotid artery	IX n	Stylohyoid ligament
	pbDGm	SPm		Pharyngeal ramus of the X n	Submandibular gland
		SHm			

MCm, middle constrictor muscle; pbDGm, posterior belly of the digastrics muscle; PGm, palatoglossus muscle; PPm, palatopharyngeus muscle; SCm, superior constrictor muscle; SGm, styloglossus muscle; SHm, stylohyoid muscle; SPm, stylopharyngeus muscle.

www.ingramcontent.com/pod-product-compliance
Lightning Source LLC
Chambersburg PA
CBHW040328220526
45473CB00009B/2608